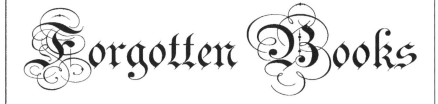

ISBN 978-0-259-99607-1
PIBN 10834811

This book is a reproduction of an important historical work. Forgotten Books uses state-of-the-art technology to digitally reconstruct the work, preserving the original format whilst repairing imperfections present in the aged copy. In rare cases, an imperfection in the original, such as a blemish or missing page, may be replicated in our edition. We do, however, repair the vast majority of imperfections successfully; any imperfections that remain are intentionally left to preserve the state of such historical works.

1 MONTH OF
FREE
READING

at

www.ForgottenBooks.com

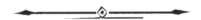

By purchasing this book you are eligible for one month membership to ForgottenBooks.com, giving you unlimited access to our entire collection of over 1,000,000 titles via our web site and mobile apps.

To claim your free month visit:
www.forgottenbooks.com/free834811

MESMERISM UNVEILED!

THE ONLY WORK EVER PUBLISHED GIVING FULL
INSTRUCTIONS HOW TO PRACTICE AND
MASTER THE ART OF PSYCHOLOGY,
OR MESMERISM.

By LESLIE J. GEE

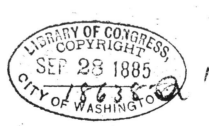

LESLIE G. DEVENPORT, PUBLISHER,
BUFFALO, N. Y.
1885.

INTRODUCTORY.

In presenting this Book to the public, it may be proper to offer some remarks relative to its origin and intent. Such as it is, however, it is respectfully submitted to the candid and deserving public, with the hope that any criticism it may excite may not be extensively distructive, but in some degree constructive. I have undertaken in this book to unfold to the enquiring public as investigators, how to practice and master the art of psychology, together with its cognates and still higher themes. It was assumed until late years, (especially by the I dont believe kind of persons) to be impossible to give any adequate exposition of this great science, but as your humble servant, I have undertaken to place it within this work so that any intelligent person can understand, practice and master it for themselves. It is in as plain language as can be used and convey my meaning. It carries the student through and explains several different modes of how to mesmerize, and gives them the most minute directions, how to operate and arrest the fluids for sickness, or to amuse. Its aim is to instruct, and the science is taught here the same as I use it in my practice on the stage.

Thanking the public for past favors, and hoping this will fill a long felt want, I remain Yours Respectfully,

LESLIE J. GEE.

MESMERISM UNVEILED.

Reader, if you have decided to undertake the study of this,-most sublime and useful of sciences, in order to gratify merely selfish desires. If you intend to use the information given in this book for your own interest alone, and to the detriment of your fellow men, let me earnestly entreat you for the good of others, and your own peace of mind to immediately destroy it. But I shall hope your motive will be pure, and your design benevolent. I am now placing in your hands a most potent agent, either for good or evil, if used for a proper purpose, with a clear appreciation of what you owe yourself and others. It will cause many to rise and call you blessed. But on the other hand, you think only of yourself, and take advantage of the multitude, and use for dishonest purposes the power I give you, (by placing it here at your command) language cannot describe the punishment you will deserve.

This study above all others must be approached with most profound feelings of reverence and awe. No trifling is excusable, no levity in place. It deals directly with the immortal part of man——the part that was created in the image of its maker. The Art of psychology or Mesmerism, gives us control over the minds and bodies of others. It teaches us how to cure deseases; gives information of the past, present and future. It places this world and the next within our comprehension, and knowledge of all beings and things within our grasp. Philosophers have reasoned and expounded. Physicians have observed and prescribed. Chemists have compounded and analyzed. Physiologists have experimented and proven, while Anatomists have dissected and laid bare the inner-most parts of man. But the part of man with which we are concerned has escaped them all. It is now fully established that somnambulists go wherever they please, without the aid of their eyes; and persons with attacks of Catalepsy, show the same peculiarity. Despine, the inspector of mineral waters at Aix, in Savoy; says of patients, "not only have I had somnambulistic patient hear by the palm of her hand, but we have seen her read without the aid of her eyes: merely with the tips of her fingers, which she passed rapidly over the page that she wished to read. At other times we have seen her select from a parcel of letters the ones she was required to pick out; also write letters and correct, on reading them over again. Always with her fingers correct the mistakes she had made. Copy one letter word for word, reading with her left elbow, while she wrote with her right hand. During these proceedings a thick pasteboard completely intercepted any visual ray that might have reached her eyes. The same phenomena was apparent at the soles of her feet; on the epigastriam and other parts of the body where a sensation of pain was produced

by mere touch. Persons who have become blind
have also been known to acquire the same power. Harriet Martineau tells of an old lady who
has been blind from her birth, yet in her sleep
she could describe the color of clothing on individuals correctly. In these cases, no doubt,
perception is as usual in the brain; but either
all the nerves of the surface have the power of
conveying impressions of light to that organ,
or some special parts of the body, as the ends
of the fingers, the occuput, or the epigastriam
assumes the office of eyes. Here are phenom-
enas showing themselves in the uninfluenced
human body, which go far towards establishing
the possibility of some of the leading principals
of the new science. Indeed, many of the feats
performed by persons in the natural somnambulistic state, rival those seen in induced somnambulism. Have we not been told by good
authority, of young ladies, finishing elegant oil
paintings in a manner far surpassing their ordinary powers, while their eyes were closed,
and they were entirely unconscious of their
acts? Do we not know of cases where men have

climbed trees and safely descended, crossed dangerous streams on narrow timbers, climb up and walk the ridge poles of a house? Either of which would have been next to impossible in their waking state. If it is possible for a person to have such acute vision in their ordinary sleep, why is it, that they should have an equal or increased power during periods of induced somnambulism? The eye, of course, is the nat ural organ of vision. But, how can persons see through obscure substances, tell what is going on in different parts of the world, or read our most secret thoughts? These are indeed very hard questions to answer, by any brinciples of Physiology or Physics. We must assume, and the facts seem to warrant the assumption, if they do not establish the conclusion, that all persons are composed of two distinct and separable parts. A body and a spirit; this last cannot be weighed, measured or acccurately defined. It is not governed by the laws that preside over matter and acts in entire independence of them. It sees through snbstances that cannot be penetrated by light. It may be acted upon without coming in contact with the body; and it has the power of discovering objects at indefinate distances, and of communicating through the body the information thus obtained to other persons. But more than this, it discovers what has happened years ago, and foretells what will occur in the future. It gives the clairvoyant subject a facility of expression, a command of language, and a store of knowledge unknown to the natural state.

Let me repeat that sublime passage on the human organism written by our most gifted dramatist: "What a piece of work is man! how noble in person, in form, in moving. How express and admirable in action. How like an angel in apprehension. How like a God. The beauty of the world; the paragon of animals."

HISTORICAL.

It is claimed by some, that the power of producing the psychologic and mesmeric state, was discovered many centuries ago; and, indeed, we have good authority to say it was known and practised in China by the Chinese, in Confucius' time, which was about 2,000 years B. C., but the first written account we have of it was contained in Confucius' writings. Confucius' writing and teachings hold the same relation to the Pagans of China, as the New Testament does to us to day. Confucius was a firm, believer in mesmerism, if we can judge by his writings. He tells us of Foo-Hung Ching, who was a celebrated mesmerist; and of his cure of the Emperior of China &c. But one of the first reliable cases heard of since that time is, that of Cordimus of Italy, who is said to have performed extraordinary cures in this way. He could bring on the mesmeric, or clairvoyant conditions at will, and thus cure himself of gout, nervous pains, &c. and prescribe remedies for himself and others. He could predict future events with precision and tell what was happening in distant countries. This was about the year 1500 A. D. Others attracted more or less attention by exhibiting similar power at intervals between that time, and the middle and eighteenth centuries. It was about this time men in different parts of Europe conceived the idea that men were sensible to the influence of magnetism.

Maxamilion Hell, Prof. of Astronomy at Vienna in the year 1772 was one of these. He advised a friend, a Physician of good standing to try if he could not cure desease by the use of the magnet. This Physician was Dr. Frederic Anthony Mesmer, whose name has since become so well known. Mesmer was well pleased with the idea, and made a large number of experiments; and succeeded so well with a great number of his patients, that he laid claim to the discovery. Prof. Hell was not satisfied with this state of affairs, and contested the discovery with Mesmer. He not only laid claim to the honor of having suggested the treatment, but he considered himself the discoverer of all the important facts made known by him who had thus become his rival. Whether public opinion went against Mesmer or not, I am not told; but he left soon after and established himself in Paris, which was then the great centre of Literature, and science. Here he met with great success, curing all kinds of bodily ailments; and all this time he used the magnets. The application of these, however, he supplanted with passes over various parts of the body, and he found the passes were as efficient as the magnets, but it is probable that after his great successes he discovered the real source of his power.

Mesmer built better than he knew. About this time the French government appointed a commission to investigate the subject. Benjamin Franklin was at the Court of Louis XV, advocating the cause of American Independance. His discoveries in electricity had already awakened the attention of the civilized world. So this plain old quaker philosopher was appointed President of the commission, which was made up of the most distinguished scientists of France. Then after a thorough investigation, during which time Mesmer practically illustrated his wondrous powers. We are told that they reported to the government that all Mesmer claimed was true, and to-day men of the highest standing are firm believers in mesmerism,

We will now devote our attention to the exploration of the mesmeric Art.

THE BENEFIT

To be derived from mesmerism, (although we use it to amuse the public, and it does amuse them. I have also mesmerized for classes in medical colleges and have instructed students the Art of Mesmerism; and as we have just mentioned, we have used it mostly to amuse, we consider this book would not be complete without a description of some of the great advantages to be derived from this useful Art.)

How often do persons who suppose they are well suddenly drop dead in a moment. How often have people retired to bed in supposed health, and yet in the morning have been found a rigid corpse either through eating too much or some other cause. The blood was suddenly propelled to the brain, and the nerves not being sufficiently braced up with galvanic fluid, collapsed, and by appoplexy instant death ensued. If these persons had been mesmerized, no such calamity would have happened. The nervous system, or the whole brain and all its ramifications would have stood the war of internal elements, and out stripped the rushing storm. In

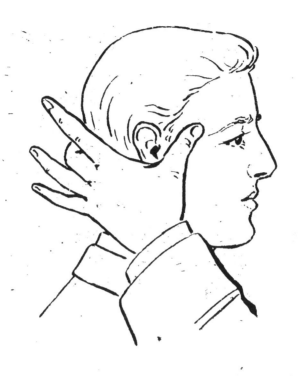

POSITION OF THE LEFT HAND,

TO BRING ON THE MESMERIC

CONDITION.

this light we see how important it is that every person, well or unwell, should be operated upon until the brain is magnetically subdued; and after its subjugation it is worth thousands of dollars to you. You are prepared for any ailments. Tooth-ache, Head-ache, Tic-dolereux, Neuralgia, with any or all these pains. Let some one mesmerise you, then wake'you up, and the pain is gone. The whole process will not take more than five minutes. If you should break an arm, or leg, have the limb mesmerized: and while it is under control you can sit and look on placidly, and see the bones set, for when under the mesmeric influence no pain is felt even during amputation; the limb can be kept in this condition until it is healed entirely. So by all means be mesmerized, that when the day of distress comes you are ready for it, and only await the mesmerist's touch.

The power of mind over matter has been recognized as a fact. Any doctor can tell you, if he has the good will of a patient, his prescriptions will work in half the time than if he has not the confidence of his patient. It is said by good authority that if a doctor has the entire confidence of his patient, and prescribes for him, when the sick person takes the bottle in his hand he feels the good effect of it, just the same as if he had taken the whole of the contents of the bottle, so strange does mind work over mind.

We have all of us in our daily vocations seen more or less Mesmerism without, perhaps, paying much attention to it. At the present time, to illustrate this, I will bring it before you. One man can subdue an unruly horse, a bull, fierce beasts, birds, serpents, or mad dogs, just with a word, look, or a stroke; whereas another man would not dare to approach either of them. This comes under the head of fascination. Our friend, Dr. Lorlard, tells me of a strong case of fascination : Three men were going along a country road; one of them stopped suddenly. The other two paying no attention to his stopping until they heard him crying at the top of his voice, " He'll bite me ! He'll bite me !" The two men made all haste to his aid, and on arriving, to their astonish ment beheld the poor fellow's eyes transfixed; and right at the edge of the road lay a large serpent half coiled, with his head high in the air, swaying from one side to the other with his forked tongue protruding, and his fire-like eyes staring at his would be victim. If it were not for the timely arrival of his companions, one of them, taking in the situation at a glance, picked up a stick from the roadside and quickly dispatched his snakeship; then the poor fellow came out of his transfixed dilemma, but not without a feeling of great weakness. He was so unstrung that he had to sit down for a short time before proceeding on his way. We have sufficient evidence of serpents doing the same to birds, rabbits, squirrels, etc., as well asmankind. A mouse put with a viper in his place of confinement has no show for life whatever. By way of experiment, one was put into a cage in New York lately. The mouse was seen to draw near the viper which lay motionless but with fixed eyes and distended mouth the mouse at length entered into its jaws and was devoured. But with the case of the man just before mentioned we would say he was in the sychological condition, for, it is said on good authority that out of every thousand people born there are forty in the psychological state, which means four out of every hundred persons born are in this state. We said and can prove that out of an audience of 1,000 persons a professional operator can tell them to close their eyes, then say authoritatively you cannot open them. There will be at least 40 that will be unable to do so, Those that are in this state are very easy to control. They can be brought under control almost by looking at them. This peculiar manifestation of the human organism has been attributed to a variety of causes by our scientific scholars. By the uninformed and ignorant, it is generally regarded as a mystery, being not unfrequently looked upon as of a magical character, the secret of which was only posessed by special individuals, only it is possible the true causes to which the psychological states are due, must remain a matter of speculation until the human organism shall be fully or more accurately understood. But the part of the ex-

planation of psychological causes explained in
this work may be depended upon as being correct; and is the pinnacle of. the knowledge
known to us to-day. But what ever the causes,
the effects are simple, and can be produced easi-
ly if the student will follow the method laid
down in this book. They are the fac simili used
by myself, and there is nothing kept from you
that can be explained in this manner. It is rea-
sonable to suppose that the human system contains two sets of nerves: motion, and sensation,
and are pervaded with fluid the same as the
veins, and other recepticals of the body are filled with appropriate liquids; and it is also rea-
sonable to admit that the internal form which
is so much more perfect than the outer, should
be connected with it, by a very refined and im-
ponderable essence. So it is by abstracting and
influencing this life essence, in the two sets of
nerves, in many and various proportions, that
the various results of mesmerism are produced.
from natural sleep, to sleep waking, sympathism,
catalepsy, interior exaltation and total separation, which is death. We know the principles

and effect of mesmerism, have a counterpart in various laws of nature. Equilibrium, attraction, renovation, development, association. No person that has ever tried it with their own hands, can deny the reality of the phenomena elicited. It has been proved, and this by Mesmer, that in every man, woman, and child born there runs through the system a mysterious fluid, by which life originates, and by which life is preserved. Controlling this fluid, life is preserved and all kinds of ailments cured. We will then perceive that the nervo vital fluid is manufactured by electricity taken into the lungs at every inspiration. It completely changes the whole brain, when that organ is in a healthy state. The nerves of this organ are of three kinds, viz: nerves of sensation, nerves of voluntary motion and the nerves of involuntary motion. I make these divisions, in order you may more clearly understand me when I am speaking of nervous action; and those three classes of nerves are all filled with nervo vital fluid, which is exactly prepared to come in contact with the human mind.

Let me now particularize. The nerves of sensation, are those by which feeling is carried to the brain. The voluntary is through which the mind gives motion to those parts of the body that are under control of the will. The involuntary nerves, are those that give motion to such parts of our system as are not under control of the will. None but the involuntary nerves pass to the heart, stomach and liver, so the heart will throb, the stomach digest its food, and the liver secrete its gall, awake or asleep, whether we will it or not. But to the lungs both the voluntary and involuntary nerves. The involuntary ones are, however, the most numerous, so that a man may hold his breath, and keep the lungs in suspension till he faints. Yet the involuntary nerves will get the mastery and restore him. Through these 3 sets of nerves the galvanic fluid is continually wasting, and passing from the whole system, mostly through the ends of our fingers and toes. It will be remembered, that in the nerves of the brain there is no blood. The blood is exclusively confined to veins and arteries, while the nerves are charged with this nervo vital fluid: a galvanic substance. Now if the veins and arteries are filled with blood; and if the nerves are fully charged with the galvanic fluid. In a word: if the circulating system and the nervous system are in perfect balance, health and firmness is the result. That I am right as to the nature of this nervous fluid. Take an animal and tie off the involuntary nerves that lead to the stomach, and digestion will instantly cease; then apply a moderate current of galvanism from a battery into the stomach, and digestion will immediately commence. This I have clearly proved, that the nervo vital fluid secreted by the brain is of a galvanic nature, and is manufactured from electricity, which we breath into the lungs every inspiration. I have also proved that this electric magnetic power is the only moter that can come in contact with mind; and is the agent by which the will contracts the muscles. Hence the conclusion, that by the concentration of the mind upon an individual, and by the action of the will. This fluid can be thrown upon another person, till his nervous system is fully changed. This is mesmerism.

THE PHENOMENA OF MESMERISM.

There are several stages or degrees, of what is called mesmeric influence, or in other words the mesmeric or psychic state envolves a variety of states having one common character, thus there is simple mesmeric drowsiness, or sleep, (COMA) or more profound sleep, or insensibility to pain. This I believe only occurs when the mesmeric coma is fully established; and most of the external senses together with the proper consciousness of external objects is rendered dormant, and the internal faculty of imagination is called into activity, without the guidance of true reason, phantasy, or that state in which the mesmerized person takes the mere suggestion of the mind of the operator to be realities. Phreno-mesmerism, are the manifestations of the phrenological sentiments and feelings, which is but another form of simple imaginative action, which causes the subject to feel what is done to the mesmerizer as if it was done to him. Mental attraction or apparent drawing of the subject, even contrary to his will. Cerebral attraction, or apparent illumination of the

brain with other forms which is called clairvoyance. We must now examine the medium by
which the mind acts on the body organization
viz: the brain and nervous system. It is common
to speak of the nervous system, constituting
the brain. The spinal marrow and nerves spring-
ing from this arrangement is true enough, as far
as it goes, but it is not sufficient for our purpose.
For examining the interior of the head it will
be found that every person has two distinct
brains. Those two brains are very different in
size and form; the upper and very large portion, and in fact occupies the greater part of the
cranium, or skull, and it is called the cerebrum.
The smaller portion is situated in the hind part
of the head, just above the spinal marrow, and
is called the cerebellum, or little brain. So we
may conclude that each of these brains has its
own specific use, and such we find to be the case;
and I shall endeavor to point out such of those
uses as bear upon the subject we are consid-
ering. My object at present not being to present you with a full view of the human brain,
but only as much as is necessary to be known

in order to comprehend the phenomenon of mesmerism. Now all the nerves by which we feel or act are called the voluntary or sensory nerves and may be said to arise either directly--from this larger portion of the brain, called the cerebrum, or indirectly from it by means of the spinal marrow, which is considered the continuation of the cerebrum in the body. The spinal marrow is composed of three distinct columns, the anterior or front column being formed of what are called moter nerves, that is, nerves that are considered in involuntary motion. The posterior column or hinder part of nerves of sensation, and the middle part of the column contains the roots of the nerves of respiration. Now we will say that if I raise my arm, I do so by muscular power communicated by nerves, having their origin in the cerebrum the same as in walking or any other action under control of the will, so all voluntary and outward actions are done by and through the medium of the cerebrum. This is one great use of the cerebrum, to originate and control the voluntary and sensory nerves. It is thus the sole medium

for external knowledge, and voluntary action
the great organ of what is called animal life.
Hence pressure on the cerebrum by paralizing
its action, suspends all sensation and capability
of motion; but the work of the cerebellum the
smaller and most curiously organized portion of
the brain is of another kind.   This is the organ
or fountain of organic life, that is of the life of
the external organs of the body, and of the
involuntary motion, and pulsations of the heart,
the circulation of the blood, and digestive action
of the stomach, and bowels, and action of the
reproductive organs, and the thousand functions performing within us, and over which our
will has no control.   All these functions are
under control of the nerves proceding directly
or indirectly from the cerebellum, or its appendages during wakefullness.   Both brains are
more or less in the state of activity, but of the
action of the larger one, the cerebrum, we are
conscious, so that our will rules in the animal
economy; but when sleep seals up our eyes,
the activity of the cerebrum ceases, and we become insensible to outward things and their

nature or the involuntary portion of the nerves centre, (that is the cerebellum) with its appendages has the entire control. But whatever produces a change in the state, in the fibre, in the cortical glands of the cerebrum, changes the state of the automatical action and produces either somnolency or wakefullness. Now let us apply ourselves to how to do this. It is my attention of laying down in this book a method that was never published before. Most all works on mesmerism lead you so far then drop you, (as it were) and after a few unsuccessful trials you get discourage and give it up; but, with my mode you cannot fail to make some impression, enough at least to encourage you to try again, but you must persevere a short time, the way I direct you. The mode I shall give you there has been paid $50 for in hundreds of cases to my knowledge to traveling professors for the same instruction, you find here. I will give all the information my limited space will permit and you can rest asured it is the same used by myself and other professors. First, I will gointo some of the other modes of mesmerizing, in which their will be four including my own.

Now let us go into the facts and give illustra-
tions of the mesmeric Phenomena and I think
we shall be able to understand something of
the mode I use when I put you in possession of
the key to the only way to bring it about; but
first I will-describe some other modes that are
called hypnotizing and chain mesmerism which
are highly-recommended by others. The simplest
visible state is what is called mesmeric sleep;
this you can produce by letting the person,
male or female gaze steadfastly on some fixed
object. This method---number one, is called
hypnotizing; but I consider the mesmeric mode
the best, where the person is susceptible of its
influence. As far as my practical experience
goes, by it only can the higher developments be
produced; but it makes no difference what
mode you use, the primary effect is on the state
of the cerebrum which by modifying the circulation of its blood-collapses in various degrees,
and thus assumes the somnolent state. Another
method---number two, is to sit your person on
a chair and take both hands in your left hand,

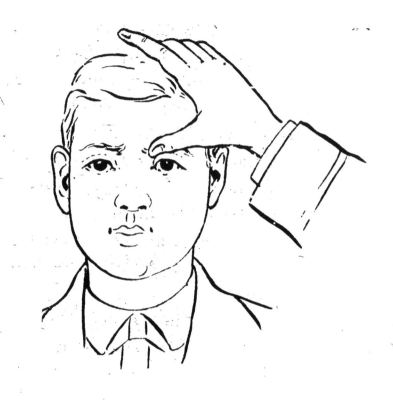

POSITION OF THE RIGHT HAND,

TO BRING ON THE MESMERIC

CONDITION.

let him or her shut their eyes, then place your right hand on the head, sitting in this position for about thirty minutes, then you may place his hands on his knees and with your hands make gentle passes from the top of his head down to his knees, and if there is any degree of mesmeric sensibility he will feel very drowsy, while other persons would be unable to open their eyes, but still are perfectly conscious all the time, then again they may go into a perfect healthy mesmeric sleep Another method is called chain mesmerism, method—number three. First get together, say four to eight persons, and form a circle, sitting firmly on their chairs; you step into the circle and endeavor to establish he communication, this is done by taking one of their hands, the left being the best, draw your thumb across the palm of the hands, incline it towards the ball of the thumb, and his will be directly over the medium nerve, which is the best nerve to get communication from. This nerve branches off at the lower part of the hand. Two large branches go to each side of the thumb and two to the index

finger, the same to the next finger and one side
of the third finger. On the other side of the
third finger is a branch of the ulner nerve and
the same in the little finger. You may try the
ulner nerve once in a while, if you wish to, this
you can do by taking the little finger between
your thumb and fore finger; but I find in my
practice the medium nerve is the best for this
kind of establishment of communication. In
drawing your thumb over the medium nerve
draw slowly six or seven times with moderate
pressure as you do so, and if the person is susceptible he will most always feel it, for a prick-
ling sensation will pass up his arm similar to
that received from a magno electric battery, a
faint shock just strong enough that you can perceive it on the subject, then let the persons sit
quietly with their hands on their knees,(for they
must be perfectly quiet, and give themselves
and their attention entirely to you,) then pass
to the next, until you have made the complete
circle then sit down yourself, and all take hold
of each others thumb; Tell them to close their
eyes or let them direct their gaze to the floor in

the centre of the circle, and sit this way at least thirty-five minutes; then if any of them fall asleep and the head drops forward you know that he has felt the soporiferous effects of attraction; and in a minute there may be more fall asleep, for this effect passes from one to another like the flash from an electric battery, then if their be more than one, sit them together, for their feelings are attracted toward each other. You may begin to mesmerize them by placing your hand upon the head (forward part) making gentle passes down the face and arms to the knees, then proceed to speak to him: ask how he likes the method, &c., if he does not wake up, continue with the passes and if he is in the true state and you continue the passes he will most always sigh; then if you want to wake him up, just say now sir I want you to wake; then clap your hands in front of his face and he will immediately wake. If you wish him to sleep he will come out of it in about one hour or perhaps sooner if he has not been under the influence before. This mode is excellent for winter evening tests for the family to determine who is the

strongest endowed operator of the family but
the wifes mesmerist should be her husband, their
relation to each other makes the ties of blood
contribute by a physical sympathy to establish
the communication. I will give you some information on how to choose subjects; then I will
proceed with method four, which is my method,
and the only one to get quick results, and is the
only one used by professional operators.

HOW TO SELECT SUBJECTS.

In the selection of subjects, it is one of the
most important things to be considered, especially for a new beginner; and if you want to
become a successful mesmerist, remember the
most accomplished mesmerist cannot mesmerize
every one as some claim. The person to be operated upon must be of a certain peculiar temperament to become a perfect subject, if he has not
this temperament all your efforts will be of no
avail. There is sufficient evidence to warrant that
every person can be mesmerized, but from
various causes, they do not all come in under it
alike. There are are some that can be controlled
in a single sitting, while others may take six

.or more of half hour each, and then fifty sittings
will not control them.   But with one more sitting they may be controlled, and make excellent
subjects. What we want to study is what per-
'sons are most susceptible, and are able to enter
the higher spheres, which mesmerism holds out.
But in my experience I find that persons with
light fine hair and light soft complexion or large
'expressive eyes, or really handsome featured,
make the best subject. Persons having these
endowments make excellent subjects, but as to
myself I have had better success with black hair
and dark eyes, they being very hard to get under
control, but once there they are excellent.   Bad
health and most kinds of deseases predispose
persons, readily to mesmerism, you must use
your own judgement to a great extent in the
selection of your subjects. A knowledge of
phrenology and physiognomy is very necessary
in the study of this art; it gives the student a
wider scope and helps you advantageously in
choosing your subject. Nevertheless, you should
choose persons younger than yourself, and persons of a different temperament, for it would be

a very difficult thing to control a person of the
same temperament as yourself. You must
persevere no matter how one may disagree
physically with any rule, perseverance must be
pre-eminent. Remember by perseverance and
patience most any man can be mesmerized.
Never mind your position in life, nor your
education, it is not necessary for you to be col-
lage bred, to become a good mesmerist, for the
very best operators are in their natural state of
uncultivated minds, method—number four.

First you must feel and put your self in a
very positive mood; then get some of your
friends allow you to operate on them, you ought
to at least have three persons to commence with;
and choose those that you feel superior to, then
you will be more or less positive to them. Why
you should have your friends is they will not be
antagonistic to you, for if they are, it will make
it up hill work for you, these persons must be
decidedly friendly to you, for you will want them
to give up entirely to you, so as to assist you in
first attempts at mesmerism, then take them into a moderately cold room for you must not try

to operate on them when they feel uncomfortably warm. Let them sit down on chairs side by
side, explain everything that is necessary and
draw their attention by talking- to them about
the benefits of mesmerism, &c. After explain-
ing this to them, then tell them to place their
feet flat upon the floor and take your left wrist in
your right hand between the thumb and index
finger, then before you proceed further ascertain
whether they have any over shoes on which are
composed of india-rubber; if they have, insist on
their taking them off, for it will interfere with
you in no small degree, by cutting off the magnetism. Also assure yourself that they have
not been drinking any intoxicating beverages;
if they have not you may then proceed, telling
them to close their eyes and let them remain
closed until you tell them to open them, then if
he can open them then let him do so; then stand
on his right front side, place the thumb of your
left hand on his right temple, and your large
finger on the back of his neck, about two inches
below the organ of amativeness, (see page 15,)
then with your right hand place your thumb on

the organ of individuality, which is located just
at the top of the nose, and the large finger on
the temple; (see page 30) then you cover four
of the proper points to bring on the first mesmeric state suddenly, or it would be of no use
to me or any other operator on the stage, or any
other place where it requires quick work. The
other point is on the top of the head which
effects the cerebrum, or large brain: the brain on
which all voluntary motion depends; then with
the large finger of the left hand you are working on the cerebrum or small brain which contains the nerves of involuntary motion, and your
thumbs are at work on the optic nerves; and
the change to be made is from the temple to the
top of the head with the right finger, and from
the back of the neck to the top of the head with
the left finger. When these changes are made
make them rather rapidly and with moderate
pressure on all points, and make about six
changes when endeavoring to charge a subject
take off your hands in a downward direction,
and at the same time say now you cannot open
your eye. It must be remembered that the down-

ward motion of the hands is the mesmeric. If you should by accident or carelessness throw your hands in an upward direction you would be likely to undo all you may have accomplished; if he succeeds in opening his eyes try him again : try him at least four times at that sitting. If you do not fasten his eyes try the next one, where you may have better success, and if you succeed in fastening his eyes the rest will be easy but until you do fasten their eyes it will not be necessary to try anything else. But fear not, you will succeed if you persevere, for you have the proper key now to the mystery of mesmerism. Do not work any more than four evenings with the same persons; if you do not succeed in fastening their eyes get some other friends to let you operate on them, and you will soon have some good subjects to work with, then you will be more successful, for when you are working on a good subject with others in the room, or on the stage it has a good effect on those that are to be worked upon when their turn comes. I have controlled persons through this influence, that I had tried several times before without any visible effects, but there is a glory in this science, though you may labor an hour each evening or day for ten or fifteen days in succestion; yet what you gain on a subject you hold until your work is complete, then you can have him do any thing you may think of, or bring him readily into the clairvoyant state which is the outcome of induced mesmerism, and at this stage you can control him or her in one or two minutes.

Be sure to keep your mind free from evil influences if you wish for success; and when you have a subject under control, do not leave him for an instant, for it effects the subject in no small degree. About three years ago in the town of M, I was instructing a young medical student in the art of mesmerism. I gave him the same information as this book contains and he was working on his first subject. His results were so surprising that he became frightened, I was in the next room and heard the commotion. I hastened out into the hallway and the young man was hastily making his retreat out of the door with a frightened look on his face. He was so thoroughly frightened that I could hardly get him to return; but I succeeded at last, and we entered the room together, when to our surprise the subject was standing in the center of the room, with eyes staring and displaying every symptom that his magnetiser may have displayed. I encouraged him to throw off his fear and stay in the room, then the subject would return to his proper condition which the did in a few minutes. It is true that the mind of the operator controls the subject. For instance, I have had some person pinch my arm, then in a short time the subject complained of being pinched, and would act the same as if it was he that really received it. When you get a good subject you may try this by way of experiment when he is under control.

We will now commence to work on the subject, if you have not succeeded in fastening his eyes yet, place your hands on the top of his head with the tips of the fingers about in the center of the head, and use a slight pressure, keep your hands this way for a few minutes. (The subjects eyes must be closed at the time.)

then change your hands as before to the back of the neck, temples, and organ of individuality, and make the same changes about six times, the same as on pages, 15 and 30. Then say, in a positive manner, you cannot open your eyes when I count three, then take your hands off. There is magnetism in the operators voice at this time, by saying you feel, see, taste, or smell &c., when I count a certain number, and it can be used to good advantage all through your working of a subject; but after controlling them once, however, it will be unnecessary, when the subjects eyes are fastened, they will appear as if they were glued together, or as if some heavy weight was on the lids holding them down, for it will be impossible for him to open them for a short time at least. You must question the subject on these points about how their eyes feel, and how impressions work on them, for I have not the space to explain them. The subject will give you valuable information and you can act accordingly. When you want to get the subject's eyes open place your fingers on his temples, and with slight pressure draw your fingers in an upward direction quickly, and say all right, or any other word you wish to use, and they will immediately open, and at the same time let your mind go with your actions. Next tell him to start his thumb going; you do it at the same time; then tell him he cannot stop it, and he will be unable to do so. Make him twirle his hands, and put a broom in his hands, and tell him he cannot let go of it, then put the broom on the floor, make a few passes down his legs and he cannot jump over it, for he will be fastened to the floor. To undo him, just touch him on the temple when he will be free, but remember your mind must go with all your work; it must be firmly set on every experiment, for the instant you let go on your mind, you lose control of your subject. Your mind is about half, and manipulation the other half that composes the practice. Then if you want him to sing, put him in a chair, tell him to close his eyes, and with your right hand place your thumb on the organ of individuality and finger on the temple, then tell him "you are an excellent singer and player, (have a broom at his side,) you will sing and play for me," when, you are saying this, draw your thumb three times down over the organ before mentioned, then say you may open your eyes and when he does, he will immediately pick up his supposed banjo and play and sing, even if he never sung before in his life. After singing, pass your finger down his left cheek, and tell him it is cold and has no feeling in it, then get a bright needle and some thread and sew his cheek and tongue. By passing the needle and thread through them, sew the left cheek; you can do this without causing the least pain to him or drawing blood, or him knowing anything about it; and if some one that saw the sewing and tell him when he is in his natural state he would not believe them, for he felt nothing nor did he bleed the slightest particle; in fact, you could fill his face full of needles and he would not know it, for the circulation of the blood is decreased, the temperature is reduced, and the nerves of voluntary motion and sensations are dormant, made so by charging the cerebrum and cerebellum with your superior force of magnetism.

The next is to put your subject in the mesmerie sleep; this is done by sitting him on a chair and tell him to go to sleep; then make passes from his forehead down to his knees untill he is fast asleep, then you may talk to him on any subject you wish to. Do not force him to open his eyes for it is very hurtful, but let him open them if he wishes to. Do not hurry him into this condition but be very gentle and kind to him; tell him to close his eyes and see what is happening in some distant country or any other place, ask him to look into some one of the company and see what they had eaten for supper. Put something over his head that he never saw before, and see if he can tell what it is, and this way of procedure he will sooner or later become clairvoyant. In making the passes always extend the fingers in the imparting of the fluid, and with the down stroke·

CATALEPSY is to make the subject's body rigid and is next to total separation, which is death. To do this stand the subject on the floor and fix your mind to what you want to do. and look him directly in the left eye; in looking at a subject (always look in his left eye,) and when working on his head, direct your gaze in the center of it, but when the subject looks at you he always looks at both of yours, and there you, have the advantage. After looking him in the eye about half a minute, place your thumb on the organ of individuality, and your left hand on the back of his neck, but before doing this make passes close to him, down his arms and legs, front and back of him down to the floor, and make the passes on his arms and legs and over the stomach, then take his head while some one else takes his feet and place him on two chairs, he will be perfectly rigid. You may stand on him without any fear of breaking the bridge thus made; do this quickly for I don't like to keep them in this state too long, their circulation being so weak, and they become quite cold; take the two chairs from under him, stand him upright. To bring him out of it it is necessary to use the most effectual way ; that is, to snap your fingers behind and in under his left ear, and when you get him complete you will be compelled to use this mode of waking them always. When you want to bring him out, especially where you make him believe the house is on fire or a snake is chasing him, or make two subjects play cards, without cards, and they get fighting over the game. You can now make them eat candles for candy, cornmeal for ice cream, castor oil for wine, cayenne pepper for sauce, or any other test you wish to put them to; but what ever you do with your subjects be kind to them, and what ever you do in this way let it be only as tests to prove the genuineness of mesmerism. Hoping I have done justice to this subject, and as I have said before, it is here for you, laid down as fully as my space will admit, and is the same as used by myself hundreds of times before audiences in most of the cities in the union; and if there is anything you cannot readily accomplish, or understand, ask the assistance of some good local mesmerist, or clairvoyant, who will put you right. If this is not at hand you can consult me either personally or by mail, at 160 SELKIRK STREET, Buffalo, N.Y., and I will do all in my power to assist you in this, the most beautiful of sciences. A few councils I wish to give you, then I have done.

Never work on a subject when he is uncomfortably warm. Always choose a cold room; the winter is the best time to operate. When a subject is too warm he will only be under your control by flashes, but when you operate on a subject his temperature will be perceptibly lowered and his circulation will be decreased.

Never handle your subject's roughly, for you are likely to throw him into convulsions; and do not try to mesmerize too rapidly. If you wish to train your subject in any class of investigation, be sure you do not force too many on him at any one time, or you will force him into the habit of guessing. Should you mesmerize any person with contagious desease, use your hands and will to throw it away from you.

Avoid mesmerizing persons as much as possible with rheumatism, unless you are mesmerizing especially for that; and use your will and hands to keep it away from you, or you will feel it in your arms or legs. But a new beginner in this art will most always feel pains in his legs and arms next morning after operating the evening before.

If when you want to operate, you do not feel strong and powerful, the following powders will help you. Purchase from your druggist five powders of five grains each of quinine, take one about two hours before you want to work, or you may take the following which I consider very good.

1 oz	-	Fluid Extract of Scullcap,
1 oz	-	" " of Valerian,
1 oz	-	" " of Catnip,
1 oz	-	" " of Coriander,
1 oz	-	Tincture of Capsicum,

Take one tea spoonful with water just before starting to operate. And remember most men can mesmerize, but some possess the power to a greater extent than others. A professional can control 40 out of one hundred. Good health is one of the first requisites. A firm energetic tranquil character together with the gift of concentrating the attention of the subject is the greatest of all aids to success.

Benevolence is a trait as valuable in a subject

as fine intellect. Male subjects are best for scientific and business purposes, female for literary and provisional.

Magnetized wands of glass or steel are very advantageous to concentrate the action upon a particular organ. For internal use magnetized water, that is done by taking a glass of water in your left hand and pointing close to the water with the fingers of the right hand, about five minutes will change it sufficiently. Magnetized water acts upon internal deseases in an astonishing manner. It carries the magnetism directly to the affected organs, the action of magnetized water is not so strong, on those who have not been magnetized.

Magnetized stockings produce a warmth to the feet which can scarcely be produced by any other means.

Clairvoyants are good for new beginners in the art, to tell them who to pick for subjects, they can tell immediately whether a person you bring to them will make a good subject under your management or not.

Nearly the most important part of a trial on a

new subject is your confident and assured
manner towards him, to give him the apprehension of your power to control him. In a little
while it will be very advantageous to you if you
make a practice of working on your subjects at
the same hour each day or night. You can impress equally as well on a person who does not
believe in mesmerism, as on one that does, it
makes no material difference how he resists
mentally, so long as he does not resist physically;
nor can subjects be dealt with harshly, for they
have double power to resist.

You must not affect to make a subject clairvoyant immediately, especially a healthy one,
for it may require a hundred sittings before you
accomplish it to your satisfaction.

The magnetizer can often impress upon his
subject a resolution for his good; and here is a
cure for intemperance or any other bad habit he
may have contracted. Have no one for magnetizer that you cannot look upon as a friend;
and be sure he is perfectly healthy, or he will ere
long communicate to you his ailments, and in-
jure himself and you also. It is always best to

know the character and principle of your magnetiser before you entrust him.

To conclude I leave you to yourself, persevere and you caunot help but succeed for Animal magnetism is a fact.

Mesmerism and clairvoyance is born of it; and IF IT BE NOT, then do no facts exist.

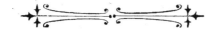